Embracing Alopecia: A Comprehensive Guide
to Understanding and Coping with Hair Loss

Hello there!

My name is Robersena Gibbs, I am a mom of four and a grandmother of two. I'm a licensed cosmetologist and a Holistic Trichology Practitioner. I am passionate about helping those who have alopecia because in 2003 my grandmother passed and the world I knew changed also. At that time, I was a mother of an 8-year-old and a 10-month-old. My youngest child's father and my best friend at that time was also gone. My stress level was at a record high. I didn't know how to cope with the grief. It negatively affected my hair. That is when my journey with alopecia began. At the age of 26, my hair started falling out. I went to seasoned hairstylists, and they couldn't help. I also visited two different dermatologists. They could not help. So I asked God why and to order my steps.

I began to help myself and others not only grow their hair back but also embrace the journey. When they would sit in my chair we would cry and talk. I would listen and provide them with different solutions. We embarked on the journey together, restored their hair, and regained their confidence. Yes, it's more than just hair to me.

In the subsequent chapters, we will explore various strategies for coping with the emotional aspects of her loss, as well as practical tips for managing and embracing alopecia in every day life. Remember, you're not alone on this journey, and there is support and guidance available to help you navigate the challenges of living with alopecia.

Disclaimer

I am not a doctor or a medical professional. The information I provided is for general informational purposes only and should not be considered as medical advice. Always consult with a qualified healthcare professional regarding any medical concerns or conditions.

Introduction

Alopecia affects many people in different ways. How one handles alopecia is critical, but all hope is not lost. This e-book is an essential guide designed to provide support, understanding, and practical advice for individuals navigating the journey of alopecia. Whether you are personally affected by alopecia or are supporting a loved one who is, this e-book aims to empower you with knowledge, strategies, and inspiration to embrace your unique beauty confidently.

Table of Contents

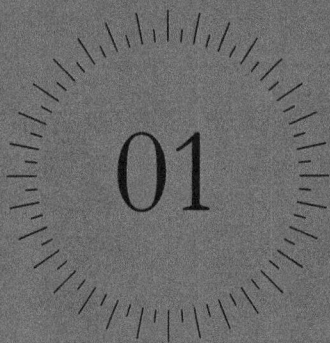

Understanding Alopecia

Understanding Alopecia

Alopecia is a condition that affects millions of people worldwide, causing variant degrees of hair loss and often carrying significant emotional and psychological implications. In this chapter, we will dive into the different types of alopecia, explore underlying causes, and shed light on the emotional impact it can have on individuals.

What is Alopecia?

Alopecia, derived from the Greek word "alopex" meaning box, refers to a medical condition characterized by the partial or complete loss of hair from areas of the body where it normally grows. While most commonly associated with hair loss on the scalp, alopecia can manifest in various forms, affecting different parts of the body, including the eyes and eyelashes. It can also affect the entire body.

Types of Alopecia

Alopecia is a general term for hair loss. There are many different types of alopecia, each with its cause and symptoms. Here are some of the most common types:

Androgenetic alopecia, also known as male pattern or female pattern baldness. Androgenetic alopecia is the most common type of hair loss, affecting both men and women. It is typically categorized by a gradual thinning of hair, often starting at the temple or crown of the head.

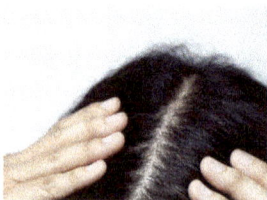

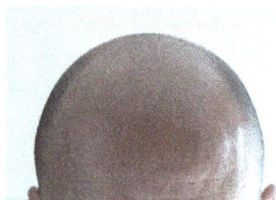

Types of Alopecia

Cicatricial alopecia: This is a type of alopecia that causes permanent hair loss. It is caused by scarring of the scalp, which destroys the hair follicles and prevents hair from growing back. There are many different causes of cicatricial alopecia, including infections, burns, and certain medical conditions.

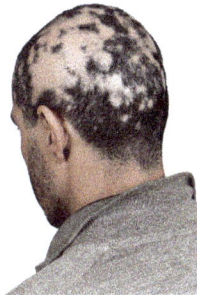

Types of Alopecia

Alopecia areata: This is an auto-immune disorder that causes sudden, patchy hair loss. It occurs when the immune system mistakenly attacks hair follicles, leading to hair loss and small round patches on the scalp.

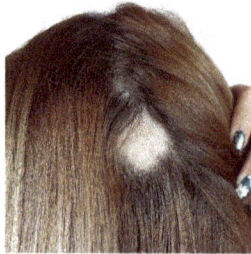

Types of Alopecia

Alopecia totalis: This is where alopecia areata progresses to involve the complete loss of hair on the scalp.

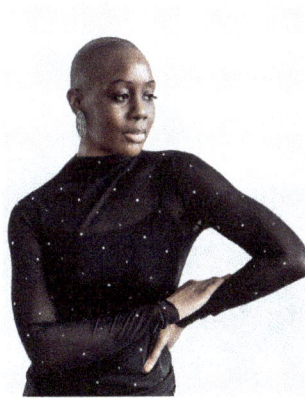

Types of Alopecia

Alopecia Universalis: Alopecia universalis is the most severe form of alopecia areata. It results in the total loss of hair on the scalp, as well as the entire body, including eyebrows, eyelashes, and other body hair.

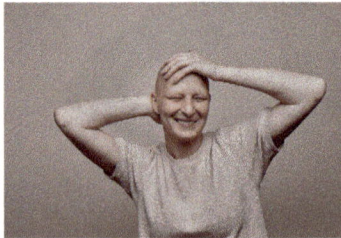

Types of Alopecia

Traction alopecia: Traction alopecia is caused by repetitive pulling or tension on the hair follicle. It is often due to hairstyles that involve tight braids, ponytails, or hair extensions. Over time, this constant pulling can lead to hair loss, particularly along the hairline.

These are just a few examples of various types of alopecia, each with unique characteristics and underlining mechanisms.

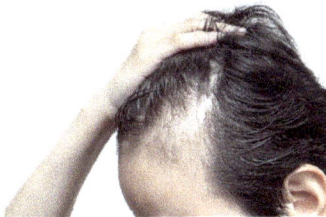

Causes and Triggers of Alopecia

The exact cause of alopecia can vary depending on the type. Several factors may contribute to its development:

- Genetics: Androgenetic alopecia, in particular, often has a strong genetic component with susceptibility to hair loss inherited from one or both parents.

- Autoimmune Factor: In the case of alopecia areata, the immune system mistakenly targets hair follicles, leading to inflammation and hair loss.

Causes and Triggers of Alopecia

- Hormonal Changes: Hormonal imbalances, such as those associated with puberty, pregnancy, or menopause, can contribute to hair loss in both men and women.

- Stress and Trauma: Emotional or physical stressors can sometimes trigger or exacerbate hair loss, particularly in individuals with a predisposition to alopecia.

- Medical Conditions and Treatments: Certain medical conditions, such as thyroid disorder and treatments like chemotherapy, can lead to temporary or permanent hair loss.

Causes and Triggers of Alopecia

Understanding the underlying causes and triggers of alopecia is crucial for both diagnosis and treatment, as it can help healthcare providers develop tailored management plans for individuals affected by the condition.

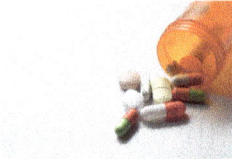

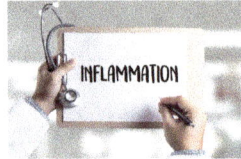

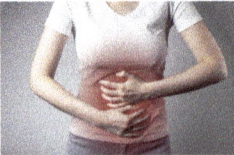

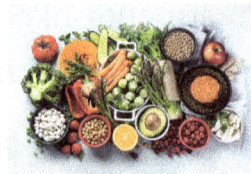

The Emotional Impact of Hair Loss

Beyond the physical symptoms, alopecia can have a profound emotional and psychological impact on those affected. The loss of hair, a defining aspect of one's appearance, can lead to feelings of self-consciousness, low self-esteem, and depression in some cases. Coping with these emotional challenges is an essential aspect of managing alopecia and promoting overall well-being.

Chapter

02

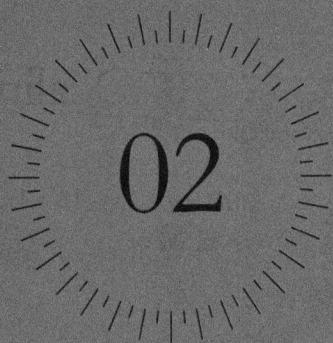

Coping With the Emotional Aspect of Hair Loss

Dealing with Hair Loss

Dealing with hair loss can be emotionally challenging, impacting one's self-esteem, confidence, and overall well-being. In this chapter, we will explore various strategies for coping with the emotional aspects of alopecia and finding confidence in your unique appearance.

Seek Support

- Join a support group: Connecting with others who are going through similar experiences can provide valuable emotional support and reassurance.
- Talk to a therapist: A mental health professional can help you process your feelings and develop coping strategies for managing the emotional impact of hair loss.

Dealing with Hair Loss

Practice Self-Compassion

- Be kind to yourself: Recognize that the experience is not your fault and that you're not alone in your struggles.
- Focus on your strength: Shift your focus from your appearance to your inequalities, talents, and accomplishments.

Challenge Negative Thoughts

- Identify and challenge negative self-talk. Replace self-critical thoughts with more balanced and compassionate statements.
- Practice gratitude: Cultivate an attitude of gratitude by focusing on the things in your life that bring you joy and fulfillment.

Dealing with Hair Loss

Experiment with Different Styles

- Embrace your baldness: Experiment with different hairstyles, including shaving your hair or rocking a buzz cut to find a look that makes you feel confident and empowered.
- Explore alternative hair options: Consider wearing wigs, hairpieces, or scarves if you prefer to cover up your hair loss temporarily.

Take Care of Yourself

- Practice self-care: Engage in activities that nourish your mind, body, and soul, such as exercising, meditation, or hobbies you enjoy.
- Prioritize your health: Focus on maintaining a healthy lifestyle, including proper nutrition, regular exercise, and sufficient sleep to support overall well-being.

Dealing with Hair Loss

Educate Others

- Educate friends and family: Help others with alopecia by sharing information and dispelling myths and misconceptions.
- Advocate for inclusivity: Encourage greater representation and awareness of alopecia in media, fashion, and beauty industries.

Embrace Your Unique Beauty

- Celebrate your uniqueness: Embrace your alopecia as a part of your identity and celebrate the beauty of diversity.
- Focus on inner beauty: Recognize that beauty comes from within and is not solely defined by external appearance.

03

Practical Tips for Managing and Embracing Alopecia in Everyday Life

Managing Alopecia

Living with alopecia presents unique challenges in daily life, from managing healthcare to navigating social situations. In this chapter, we will explore practical tips and strategies for managing and embracing alopecia in various aspects of everyday life.

Hair Care

- Keep your scalp and hair moisturized.
- Use gentle cleansers and moisturizers to keep your scalp healthy and prevent dryness or irritation.
- Protect your scalp from the sun: Wear sunscreen or a hat to protect your scalp from sunburn, especially if you have alopecia universals.

Managing Alopecia

Styling

- Experiment with different styling techniques: Get creative with scarves, hats, or head wraps to accessorize your look and express your style. Opt for maintenance hairstyles.

Makeup and Skincare

- Features with makeup: Experiment with makeup techniques to accentuate your eyes, lips, and other facial features and boost your confidence.
- Take care of your skin: Keep your skin healthy and glowing by following a regular skincare routine, including cleansing, moisturizing, and protecting your skin from the sun.

Managing Alopecia

Social Situations

- Communicate your preferences: Communicate your preferences regarding questions or comments about your alopecia to friends, family, and acquaintances.
- Practice self-assertiveness: Assertively set boundaries and advocate for yourself and social situations to ensure that your needs and feelings are respected.

Professional Settings

- Be confident in professional settings: Focus on your skills, expertise, and qualifications rather than worrying about your appearance in professional settings.
- Educate colleagues and employees: Inform them about any accommodations or support you need in the workplace.

Managing Alopecia

Relationships and Dating

- Be open and honest: Be open and honest about your alopecia when forming new relationships or dating, and share information as you feel comfortable.
- Focus on mutual connections: Look for partners who appreciate and value you for who you are beyond your appearance and support you in embracing your alopecia.

By implementing these practical tips and strategies, you can navigate the challenges of living with alopecia with confidence and grace. You will be able to embrace your unique beauty and live life to the fullest. Remember, alopecia does not define you. It is just one aspect of your identity, and you are so much more than your hair.

Diagnosis and Treatment Options for Alopecia

Diagnosing Alopecia

Diagnosing alopecia typically involves a combination of medical history, physical examination, and sometimes, additional tests to determine the underlying cause and extent of hair loss. Here are some common diagnostic methods:

- Medical History: Your healthcare provider will inquire about your medical history, including any family history of hair loss, recent illness or treatments, and any medication you may be taking.
- Physical Examination: A thorough physical exam of the scalp, hair, and other areas of the body affected by hair loss can provide valuable insight into the pattern and severity of alopecia.

Diagnosing Alopecia

- Pull Test: During a pull test, your healthcare provider gently pulls on a small section of hair to assess how much hair comes out. An increased number of hair being pulled out may indicate active hair shedding.
- Scalp Biopsy: In this case, a scalp biopsy may be performed to obtain a small sample of skin tissue for microscopic examination. This can help identify any underlying inflammatory or auto-immune processes contributing to hair loss.
- Blood Tests: Blood tests may be ordered to check for underlying medical conditions or hormonal imbalances that could be contributing to hair loss, such as thyroid disease or androgen level.

Treatment for Alopecia

Treatment options for alopecia vary depending on the type, severity, and underlying causes of her loss. While some treatments aim to manage symptoms and slow hair loss progression, others may target the underlying cause or stimulate hair growth. Here are some common treatment options.

- Medications: You can utilize topic solutions applied to the scalp.
- Hair Transplantation Scalp
  Micro pigmentation.
- Wigs and Hairpieces: For individuals experiencing significant hair loss, wigs, hairpieces, and hair extensions offer a non-invasive and versatile solution to conceal hair loss and enhance appearances.

Treatment for Alopecia

It is essential to consult with a healthcare professional, Trichologist, or dermatologist to determine the most appropriate treatment approach. Based on your individual needs, preferences, and the specific type of alopecia you have. Additionally, some individuals may benefit from a combination of treatments to achieve optimum results. Keep in mind that results may vary, and it may take time to see noticeable improvements in hair growth or appearance.

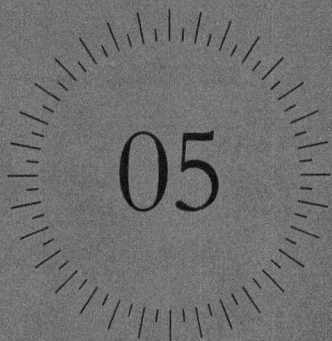

Embracing Change and Self-Discovery

Embrace the Journey

Living with alopecia can be a transformative journey that challenges perceptions of beauty, identity, and self-worth. In this chapter, we will explore the process of embracing change and self-discovery while navigating the realities of hair loss.

Embrace the Journey

Redefining Beauty Standards

One of the most profound aspects of living with alopecia is the opportunity to challenge conventional beauty standards and redefine what it means to be beautiful. Rather than adhering to narrow ideals dictated by society, individuals with alopecia have the chance to embrace their unique appearance and celebrate the diversity of human beauty. By shifting the focus from external appearance to inequalities, such as kindness, compassion, and resilience, it becomes possible to cultivate a deep sense of self-worth and confidence.

Embrace the Journey

Coping with Emotional Challenges

Embracing change involves confronting the emotional challenges of hair loss, including feelings of grief, self-doubt, and insecurity. It's normal to experience a range of emotions when faced with the realities of alopecia, but it's essential to acknowledge and process these feelings rather than suppressing them. Seeking support from loved ones, joining support groups, or speaking with a therapist are ways to work through emotions. Individuals with alopecia can gain valuable insight and coping strategies to navigate the emotional roller coaster of hair loss.

Embrace the Journey

Building Self-Confidence and Resilience

Embracing alopecia requires cultivating self-confidence and resilience in the face of adversity. Rather than allowing hair loss to define a sense of self-worth, individuals with alopecia can focus on their strengths, talents, and accomplishments. By setting goals, challenging themselves, and stepping outside of their comfort zones, they can be resilient and develop a strong sense of self-efficiency. Through perseverance and determination, individuals with alopecia can overcome obstacles and thrive in all aspects of life.

Sharing Your Journey

One of the most powerful ways to embrace change with alopecia is by sharing your journey with others. By being honest about your experiences, you can inspire and empower others who may be going through similar challenges. Whether through social media, support groups, or community events, sharing your story can help raise awareness, reduce stigma, and foster a sense of connection and belonging. Individuals with alopecia can find strength and validation in their shared experiences by connecting with others and building supportive networks.

Embracing Your Unique Identity

Ultimately, embracing alopecia is about embracing your unique identity and celebrating what makes you truly special. Rather than viewing hair loss as a limitation, individuals with alopecia can see it as an opportunity for self-expression and authenticity. By embracing their baldness with pride and confidence, they can inspire others to embrace their uniqueness and live authentically. Through self-discovery and self-acceptance, individuals with alopecia can unlock their full potential and lead fulfilling and meaningful lives.

In conclusion, embracing change in self-discovery with alopecia is a transformative journey that requires courage, resilience, and self-compassion. By challenging beauty standards concerning emotional challenges, building self-confidence, sharing your journey, and embracing your unique identity, you can navigate the realities of hair loss with grace and dignity. Remember, alopecia does not define you. It is just one aspect of your identity, and you are so much more than your hair.

Chapter

06

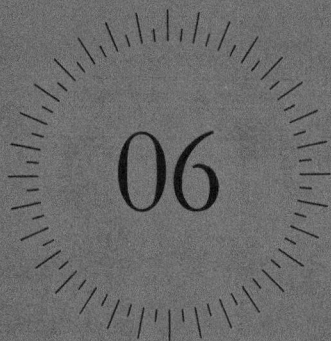

Thriving With Alopecia

Thriving with alopecia is not just about accepting hair loss. It's about embracing your unique beauty, finding and enjoying life's blessings, and pursuing your dreams with confidence. In this chapter, we will explore the transformative journey of thriving with alopecia and celebrate the resilience, strength, and courage of individuals who refuse to let hair loss define them.

Success Stories and Inspirational Journeys

Some of the most powerful aspects of thriving with alopecia are in the stories of individuals who have not only accepted their hair loss but have thrived despite it. Whether through personal anecdotes, testimonials, or interviews. Learning from the experiences of others can provide valuable insight. It can also provide inspiration and encouragement on your journey. Celebrating the success of those who have come before, you can gain perspective, hope, and motivation to pursue your dreams.

Setting Goals and Pursuing Dreams

Thriving with alopecia involves setting goals, pursuing passions, and living life to the fullest. Rather than allowing hair loss to hold you back, use it as a catalyst for growth and transformation. Whether it's by pursuing a career, traveling the world, or starting a family. Don't let alopecia stand in the way of your dreams. By setting goals, taking action, and persevering in the faith of challenges. You can create a life filled with purpose, fulfillment, and joy.

Finding Joy and Fulfillment Beyond Appearance

Thriving with alopecia requires shifting the focus from external appearance to inner fulfillment and happiness. Instead of seeking validation and approval from others, focus on cultivating joy, gratitude, and contentment from within. It could be spending time with loved ones, pursuing happiness, or practicing acts of kindness. Find activities that bring you joy and fulfillment independent of your appearance. By nurturing your inner well-being and finding happiness in the present moment, you can experience true fulfillment and live a life of abundance.

Cultivating Gratitude and Embrace Life's Blessings

Thriving with alopecia involves cultivating gratitude for the blessings in your life, even in the face of adversity. Rather than dwelling on what you've lost, focus on what you have and express gratitude for the abundance that surrounds you. Focus on your health, relationship, or personal achievements. Take time to appreciate the blessings in your life.

By shifting your perspective and focusing on the positives, you can transform challenges into opportunities for growth and find beauty in every moment.

Conclusion

Thriving with alopecia is a transformative journey of self-discovery, resilience, and empowerment. By celebrating your unique beauty, pursuing your passion, finding joy beyond appearance, and cultivating gratitude for life's blessings, you can thrive despite hair loss and live a life filled with purpose, fulfillment, and happiness. Always remember that alopecia does not define you. God says you are fearfully and wonderfully made.

Document your Process

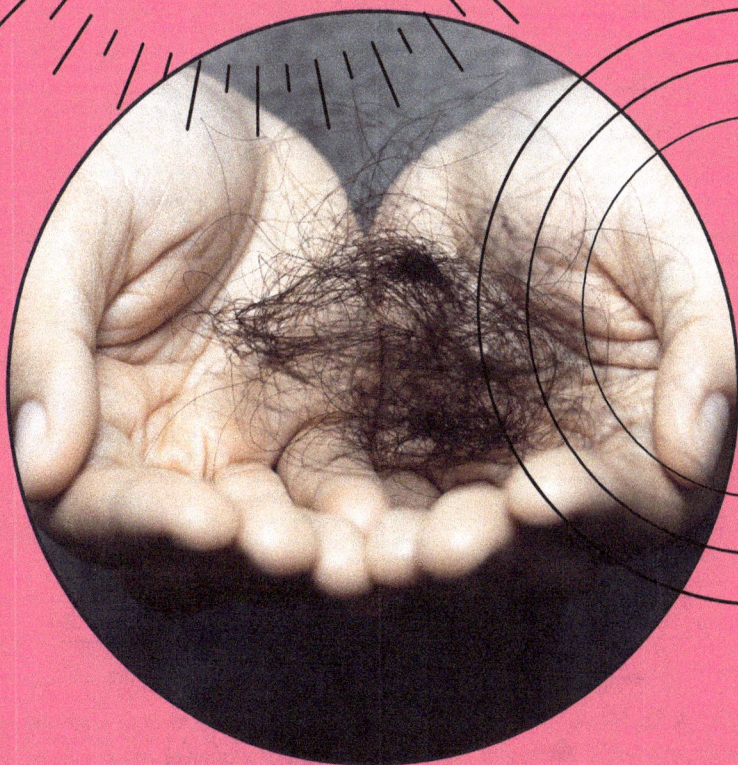

Date_____

Today I am feeling:

_____
_____
_____
_____
_____
_____
_____
_____
_____
_____
_____
_____
_____

I can be encouraged because:

_____
_____
_____
_____
_____
_____
_____
_____
_____
_____
_____
_____
_____

For I know the plans I have for you," declares the Lord, "plans to prosper you and not to harm you, plans to give you hope and a future.
Jeremiah 29:11 NIV

Date_____

Today I am feeling:

_____
_____
_____
_____
_____
_____
_____
_____
_____
_____
_____
_____
_____

I can be encouraged because:

_____
_____
_____
_____
_____
_____
_____
_____
_____
_____
_____
_____
_____

For you created my inmost being; you knit me together in my mother's womb.
Psalms 139:13 NIV

Date_____

Today I am feeling:

_____
_____
_____
_____
_____
_____
_____
_____
_____
_____
_____
_____
_____
_____

I can be encouraged because:

_____
_____
_____
_____
_____
_____
_____
_____
_____
_____
_____
_____
_____
_____

I praise you because I am fearfully and wonderfully made; your works are wonderful, I know that full well.
Psalms 139:14 NIV

Date_____

Today I am feeling:

_____
_____
_____
_____
_____
_____
_____
_____
_____
_____
_____
_____
_____
_____

I can be encouraged because:

_____
_____
_____
_____
_____
_____
_____
_____
_____
_____
_____
_____
_____

*My frame was not hidden from you when I was made in the secret place,
when I was woven together in the depths of the earth.
Psalms 139:15 NIV*

Date_____

Today I am feeling:

_____
_____
_____
_____
_____
_____
_____
_____
_____
_____
_____
_____
_____

I can be encouraged because:

_____
_____
_____
_____
_____
_____
_____
_____
_____
_____
_____
_____
_____

Your eyes saw my unformed body; all the days ordained for me were written in your book before one of them came to be.
Psalms 139:16 NIV

Date_____

Today I am feeling:

_____

_____

_____

_____

_____

_____

_____

_____

_____

_____

_____

_____

_____

_____

I can be encouraged because:

_____

_____

_____

_____

_____

_____

_____

_____

_____

_____

_____

_____

_____

Rather, it should be that of your inner self, the unfading beauty of a gentle and quiet spirit, which is of great worth in God's sight.
1 Peter 3:4 NIV

Date_____

Today I am feeling:

_____
_____
_____
_____
_____
_____
_____
_____
_____
_____
_____
_____
_____

I can be encouraged because:

_____
_____
_____
_____
_____
_____
_____
_____
_____
_____
_____
_____
_____

The eyes of the Lord are everywhere,
keeping watch on the wicked and the good.
Proverbs 15:3 NIV

Date_____

Today I am feeling:

_____
_____
_____
_____
_____
_____
_____
_____
_____
_____
_____
_____
_____

I can be encouraged because:

_____
_____
_____
_____
_____
_____
_____
_____
_____
_____
_____
_____

You are altogether beautiful, my darling;
there is no flaw in you.
Song of Songs 4:7 NIV

Date_____

Today I am feeling:

_____
_____
_____
_____
_____
_____
_____
_____
_____
_____
_____
_____
_____

I can be encouraged because:

_____
_____
_____
_____
_____
_____
_____
_____
_____
_____
_____
_____

All glorious is the princess within her chamber;
her gown is interwoven with gold.
Psalm 45:13 NIV

Date_____

Today I am feeling:

_____
_____
_____
_____
_____
_____
_____
_____
_____
_____
_____
_____
_____

I can be encouraged because:

_____
_____
_____
_____
_____
_____
_____
_____
_____
_____
_____
_____
_____

Don't you know that you yourselves are God's temple and that God's Spirit dwells in your midst?
1 Corinthians 3:16 NIV

Date_____

Today I am feeling:

_____
_____
_____
_____
_____
_____
_____
_____
_____
_____
_____
_____
_____
_____

I can be encouraged because:

_____
_____
_____
_____
_____
_____
_____
_____
_____
_____
_____
_____
_____

She is clothed with strength and dignity;
she can laugh at the days to come.
Proverbs 31: 25 NIV

Date_____

Today I am feeling:

_____
_____
_____
_____
_____
_____
_____
_____
_____
_____
_____
_____
_____
_____

I can be encouraged because:

_____
_____
_____
_____
_____
_____
_____
_____
_____
_____
_____
_____
_____

Your beauty should not come from outward adornment, such as elaborate hairstyles and the wearing of gold jewelry or fine clothes. Rather, it should be that of your inner self, the unfading beauty of a gentle and quiet spirit, which is of great worth in God's sight.

Date_____

Today I am feeling:

_____
_____
_____
_____
_____
_____
_____
_____
_____
_____
_____
_____
_____
_____

I can be encouraged because:

_____
_____
_____
_____
_____
_____
_____
_____
_____
_____
_____
_____
_____

But seek first his kingdom and his righteousness, and all these things will be given to you as well.
Matthew 6:33 NIV

Date_____

Today I am feeling:

_____
_____
_____
_____
_____
_____
_____
_____
_____
_____
_____
_____
_____
_____

I can be encouraged because:

_____
_____
_____
_____
_____
_____
_____
_____
_____
_____
_____
_____
_____

"Dear friends, now we are children of God, and what we will be has not yet been made known. But we know that when Christ appears, we shall be like him, for we shall see him as he is."
1 John 3:2 NIV

Date_____

Today I am feeling:

_____
_____
_____
_____
_____
_____
_____
_____
_____
_____
_____
_____
_____

I can be encouraged because:

_____
_____
_____
_____
_____
_____
_____
_____
_____
_____
_____
_____
_____

And, "I will be a Father to you, and you will be my sons and daughters,
says the Lord Almighty."
2 Corinthians 6:18 NIV

Date_____

Today I am feeling:

_____
_____
_____
_____
_____
_____
_____
_____
_____
_____
_____
_____
_____
_____

I can be encouraged because:

_____
_____
_____
_____
_____
_____
_____
_____
_____
_____
_____
_____

"Come to me, all you who are weary and burdened, and I will give you rest. Take my yoke upon you and learn from me, for I am gentle and humble in heart, and you will find rest for your souls. For my yoke is easy and my burden is light."
Matthew 11:28-30 NIV

Date_____

Today I am feeling:

_____
_____
_____
_____
_____
_____
_____
_____
_____
_____
_____
_____
_____

I can be encouraged because:

_____
_____
_____
_____
_____
_____
_____
_____
_____
_____
_____
_____
_____

"The Lord will vindicate me; your love, Lord, endures forever—
do not abandon the works of your hands."
Psalms 138:8 NIV

Date_____

Today I am feeling:

_____
_____
_____
_____
_____
_____
_____
_____
_____
_____
_____
_____
_____

I can be encouraged because:

_____
_____
_____
_____
_____
_____
_____
_____
_____
_____
_____
_____
_____

"So God created mankind in his own image, in the image of God he created them;
male and female he created them."
Genesis 1:27 NIV